5 INGREDIENTS   LOW CALORIE   NO FUSS

The Simple

5 Ingredient *Skinny* SLOW COOKER

 CookNation

The Simple 5 Ingredient Skinny Slow Cooker Recipe Book
5 Ingredients, Low Calorie, No Fuss.

ISBN: 978-1-912155-87-3

Disclaimer

Contents

Skinny Slow Cooker Fish Dishes   51

Skinny Slow Cooker Vegetable & Vegetarian Dishes 61

Skinny Slow Cooker Soups   73

Skinny Slow Cooker & Treats & Puddings   85

Other CookNation Titles   96

Introduction

Anyone with a busy life knows that meal times can be tough. You may be a parent who needs to feed the family, single with a busy demanding job, a student on a budget or just simply out of fresh ideas to keep yourself on track.

Thankfully there's a solution that will help. The slow cooker is the lifesaver you've been looking for. With our recipes that contain only 5 ingredients, you can prep meals every day in minutes and leave your slow cooker to do the work. For those watching their waistline you can take comfort in the fact that each delicious recipe is calorie counted and falls below either 200, 300, 400, 500 and 600 calories per serving.

When life takes over, often poor food choices are made but it needn't be that way. Our recipes are no fuss, low calorie and really do only need 5 ingredients to deliver a delicious, nutritious meal that will allow you stay on track with your weight loss efforts.

Wherever possible our recipes try to use fresh ingredients and balance the meal with protein, fat and good carbs however some dishes may require side servings of salad or rice for example. We've included some guidance throughout the book. Remember though if you are counting your calories then any additional side dishes will increase your calorie intake.

Most of our recipes serve either 4 or 6 making it them perfect for family meal times or to freeze for yourself for another day.

Many recipes make use of hero ingredients such as pesto or curry paste that are packed full of flavour and will really intensify the taste of your meal - they are also great time savers when you're prepping. Fresh herbs are another way to get great flavours into your meals. Try buying the potted varieties from your supermarket - they will last a lot longer than the prepared packs or even better, grow your own on a sunny window ledge.

When choosing your meat, try to be selective and, if you can, opt for cuts from organic, grass fed animals. You can often choose cheaper cuts of meat for the slow cooker as the process of cooking over a number of hours intensifies flavour and tenderises the meat. Similarly with dairy products, organic is better not just for the welfare of the animal from which it came but also because you will notice the difference in flavour. Fish should also be as fresh as you can source it.
Buying organic can cost more so if you are on a budget it is not essential for our recipes.

You will notice at first glance that many recipes appear to use more than 5 ingredients. This is because most recipes require key staples to cook. These items should always be in your store cupboard – you will most likely already have them:

- Salt & pepper
- Cooking oil spray
- Olive Oil
- Coconut oil
- Stock (Chicken, Beef, Vegetable, Fish)

Our skinny low calorie recipes are the pathway to stress-free, simple, quick and easy meal times. The combination of just 5 ingredients each time will deliver flavoursome dishes with minimum prep while your slow cooker works its magic while you get on with your life.

Preparation

All of the recipes take no longer than 10-15 minutes to prepare. Browning the meat will make a difference to the taste of your recipe but if you really don't have the time, don't worry. Similarly sautéing ingredients like onions or garlic can add sweetness or intensity to a dish. If time isn't on your side you don't need to do this but for the days when you have an extra few moments to spare, give it a try and see if you can taste the difference.

All meat and vegetables should be cut into even sized pieces.
Meat generally cooks faster than vegetables, although root vegetables can take
All meat should be trimmed of visible fat and the skin removed.

Low Cost

Slow cooking is ideal for cheaper meat cuts. The 'tougher' cuts used in this collection of recipes are transformed into meat which melts-in-your-mouth and helps to keep the costs down. We've also made sure not to include too many one-off ingredients that are used for a single recipe and never used again. All the herbs and spices listed can be used in multiple recipes throughout the book.

Nutrition

While we have tried to balance our recipes as much as possible, inevitable with just 5 ingredients this isn't always possible.

If you are following a diet, it is important to balance your food between proteins, good carbs, dairy, fruit and vegetables. Try to select differently recipes throughout the week to hit each of the main food groups and supplement your meals accordingly to stay healthy.

Even on a diet you should be aiming to include the following food groups into your meals:

- **Protein**. Keeps you feeling full and is also essential for building body tissue. Good protein sources come from meat, fish and eggs.

- **Carbohydrates.** Carbs are generally high in calories, which make them difficult to include in a calorie limiting diet. Carbs are a good source of energy for your body as they are converted more easily into glucose (sugar), providing energy. Try to eat 'good carbs' which are high in fibre and nutrients e.g. whole fruits and veg, nuts, seeds, whole grain cereals, beans and legumes.

- **Dairy.** Dairy products provide you with vitamins and minerals. Cheeses can be high in calories but other products such as fat free Greek yoghurt, crème fraiche and skimmed milk are all good.

- **Fruit & Vegetables.** Eat your five a day. There is never a better time to fill your 5 a day quota. Not only are fruit and veg very healthy, they also fill up your plate and are ideal snacks when you are feeling hungry.

Our Skinny Recipes

The recipes in this book are all low calorie dishes serving 4-6, which makes it easier for you to monitor your overall daily calorie intake as well as those you are cooking for. The recommended daily calories are approximately 2000 for women and 2500 for men.

Broadly speaking, by consuming the recommended levels of calories each day you should maintain your current weight. Reducing the number of calories (a calorie deficit) will result in losing weight. This happens because the body begins to use fat stores for energy to make up the reduction in calories, which in turn results in weight loss. We have already counted the calories for each dish making it easy for you to fit this into your daily eating plan whether you want to lose weight, maintain your current figure or are just looking for some great-tasting, skinny slow cooker meals.

Many of our recipes offer an optional serving suggestion which are helpful when cooking for family or friends. For example serving with rice, pasta or potatoes. These are additional servings that are not included in the recipe calorie count. If you choose to include these please be aware that you will need to allow for the additional calories if you are on a diet.

I'm Already On A Diet. Can I Use These Recipes?

Yes of course. All the recipes can be great accompaniments to many of the popular calorie-counting diets. We all know that sometimes dieting can result in hunger pangs, cravings and boredom from eating the same old foods day in and day out. Our skinny slow cooker recipes provide filling meals that should satisfy you for hours afterwards.

I Am Only Cooking For One. Will This Book Work For Me?

Yes. We would recommend following the method for 4-6 servings then dividing and storing the rest in single size portions for you to use in the future. Most of the recipes will freeze well. Allow your slow cooked meals to cool to room temperature before refrigerating or freezing. When ready to defrost, allow to thaw in a fridge overnight then at room temperature for a few hours depending on the size of portion. Reheat thoroughly.

Portion Sizes

The majority of recipes are for 4-6 servings. The calorie count is based on one serving. It is important to remember that if you are aiming to lose weight using any of our skinny recipes, the size of the portion that you put on your plate will significantly affect your weight loss efforts. Filling your plate with over-sized portions will obviously increase your calorie intake and hamper your dieting efforts.

It is important with all meals that you use a correct sized portion, which generally is the size of your clenched fist. This applies to any side dishes of vegetables and carbs too.

About Your Slow Cooker

- Our recipes have been tested using a 6.5 litre capacity slow cooker. You may need to adjust quantities and cooking times to suit your own appliance.
- All cooking times are a guide. Make sure you get to know your own slow cooker so that you can adjust timings accordingly.
- Read the manufacturers operating instructions as appliances can vary. For example, some recommend preheating the slow cooker for 20 minutes before use whilst others advocate switching on only when you are ready to start cooking.
- Slow cookers do not brown-off meat. While not always necessary, if you do prefer to brown your meat you must first do this in a pan with a little low calorie cooking spray.
- A spray of one calorie cooking oil in the cooker before adding ingredients will help with cleaning or you can buy slow cooker liners.
- Don't be tempted to regularly lift the lid of your appliance while cooking. The seal that is made with the lid on is all part of the slow cooking process. Each time you do lift the lid you will need to increase the cooking time.
- Removing the lid at the end of the cooking time can be useful to thicken up a sauce by adding additional cooking time and continuing to cook without the lid on. On the other hand if perhaps a sauce it too thick removing the lid and adding a little more liquid can help.
- Always add hot liquids to your slow cooker, not cold.
- Do not overfill your slow cooker.
- Allow the inner dish of your slow cooker to completely cool before cleaning. Any stubborn marks can usually be removed after a period of soaking in hot soapy water.
- Be confident with your cooking. Feel free to use substitutes to suit your own taste and don't let a missing herb or spice stop you making a meal - you'll almost always be able to find something to replace it.

About CookNation

CookNation is the leading publisher of innovative and practical recipe books for the modern, health conscious cook.

CookNation titles bring together delicious, easy and practical recipes with their unique approach - easy and delicious, no-nonsense recipes - making cooking for diets and healthy eating fast, simple and fun. With a range of #1 best-selling titles - from the innovative 'Skinny' calorie-counted series, to the 5:2 Diet Recipes collection - CookNation recipe books prove that 'Diet' can still mean 'Delicious'!

To browse all CookNation's recipe books visit *www.bellmackenzie.com*

Skinny
SLOW COOKER
meat dishes

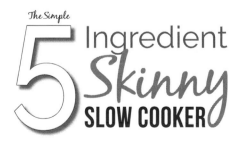

The Simple
5 Ingredient
Skinny
SLOW COOKER

Coriander Chicken

2 x 225g/8oz jars salsa

Juice of 1 fresh lime, halved and squeezed

1 tbsp taco seasoning

3 tbsp fresh coriander, chopped

1.35kg/3lbs chicken breasts, halved lengthwise

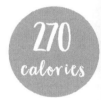

270 calories

- In your slow cooker, mix together the salsa, lime juice, taco seasoning and coriander. Drop in the chicken breasts and coat them with the salsa mixture.

- Cover, and cook on High for about 4 hours, or on Low for 6-8 hours, until the chicken is very tender.

- Once cooked, use 2 forks to shred the chicken.

- Serve hot, with steamed rice, garnished with fresh slices of lime or slivers of red chilli.

Reserve a little fresh coriander to sprinkle on top when serving.

Hoisin Chicken

Non-stick vegetable cooking spray

1.5kg/3½lbs chicken thighs, skinned

Salt & pepper

120ml/½ cup hoisin sauce

225g/8oz fresh broccoli, broken into small florets

225g/8oz fresh carrots, peeled & sliced diagonally

200g/7oz cooked rice

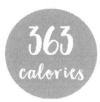

363 calories

- Spray your slow cooker with non-stick oil. Add the chicken thighs. Season well with salt and pepper and pour the hoisin sauce over the top.

- Cover and cook on Low for 5 hours or on High for 2½ hours.

- Stir in the broccoli and carrots. Cook on High for another 30-40 minutes.

- Stir in the cooked rice. Heat, covered, for another few minutes, and then serve hot in warmed Chinese style bowls.

For speed, substitute a frozen mix of vegetables for the fresh broccoli and carrots.

Sweet and Sharp BBQ Chicken

1.1kg/2½lbs chicken drumsticks, skinned

250ml/1 cup barbecue sauce

3 tbsp apricot preserve

2 tsp English mustard

200g/7oz cooked rice

521 calories

- Throw the chicken into your slow cooker.

- In a bowl, mix together the barbecue sauce, apricot preserve and mustard. Pour the sauce over the chicken.

- Cover and cook on Low for 6 to 8 hours or on High for 3 to 4 hours.

- Stir in the rice, cover, and cook for another 5 minutes to let the rice absorb the flavours.

- Serve on warmed plates, garnished with slices of fresh apricot.

Delicious also with peach or plum preserve instead of apricot.

Chicken with Sweet Potatoes

1 onion, peeled & finely chopped

2 medium sweet potatoes, peeled & diced

½ tsp smoked paprika

Salt and freshly ground black pepper

250ml/1 cup low fat chicken stock

675g/1½lb chicken thighs, skinned

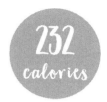

232 calories

- Add the onions and sweet potatoes into your slow cooker. Add half the paprika and a good grinding of black pepper. Pour in the chicken stock.

- In a small bowl combine the rest of the paprika with some salt and pepper. Rub the mixture onto the chicken thighs and add them to the slow cooker.

- Cover and cook on Low for about 3½-4 hours, until the chicken is well-cooked and the sweet potatoes are tender.

- Adjust the seasoning and serve hot, with a few drops of balsamic vinegar on each serving.

Use unsmoked paprika if you prefer.

Mustard and Maple Syrup Chicken

3 large skinless chicken breasts, halved

120ml/½ cup maple syrup

2 tbsp Dijon mustard

2 tbsp tapioca

200g/7oz cooked rice

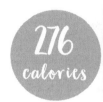

276 calories

- Place the chicken breasts in your slow cooker.

- In a small bowl, mix together the maple syrup, mustard and tapioca, then pour it over the chicken.

- Cover and cook on Low for 3-4 hours or until the chicken is tender. Stir in the rice, re-cover and leave the rice to absorb the flavours for a few minutes.

- Serve on warmed plates.

For a stronger flavour, use English instead of Dijon mustard.

Hawaiian Chicken

6 rashers of back bacon

Salt & freshly ground black pepper

6 boneless, skinless chicken thighs

1 onion, peeled & finely chopped

225g/8oz pineapple, crushed & drained

250ml/1 cup barbecue sauce

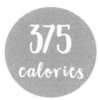

375 calories

- Cut three of the bacon strips in half and fry. Remove them from the pan before they're crisp, and drain them on kitchen towel and use these on top of the chicken.

- Season the chicken thighs and place them in your slow cooker. Top each thigh with a piece of bacon. Add the onion, pineapple and barbecue sauce.

- Cover and cook on Low for about 5 hours, or until the chicken is tender. Fry the remaining bacon until crisp. Cool it and crumble it.

- Serve the chicken on warm plates and scatter some crumbled bacon over each serving.

Tinned or fresh pineapple works for this simple sweet recipe.

Chicken Salsa

1 large onion, peeled & thinly sliced

900g/2lb skinless chicken breasts

2 peppers de-seeded & finely sliced

450g/16oz salsa

½ tsp salt

Juice of 1 fresh lime

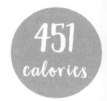

451 calories

- Throw the chicken into your slow cooker. Add the onion, peppers, salsa and salt, and stir it all up.

- Cover and cook on High for 4 hours or Low for at least 6, until the chicken is very tender.

- When it's cooked use two forks to shred the chicken.

- Add the lime juice and adjust the seasoning. Serve with tortillas, topped with slices of avocado and lime, and a dollop of sour cream.

Choose spicy or mild salsa to suit your own taste.

Chicken and Kale with Pasta

450g/1lb skinless chicken breasts or thighs

2 large potatoes, peeled & cubed

140g/4½oz fresh kale, stems removed, finely chopped

1lt/4 cups chicken stock

Salt & pepper

2 tsp Italian seasoning

200g/7oz pasta shells

385 calories

- Add all the ingredients except the pasta to your slow cooker. Stir them together, then cover and cook on High for about 3½ hours or on Low for 6, or until the potatoes are tender and the chicken is cooked through and very tender.

- Using two forks, shred the chicken. Add the pasta shells, and a little water or stock if necessary, then cook for another 30 minutes or until the pasta is tender.

- Adjust the seasoning, and serve hot, garnished with basil leaves and a few drops of good olive oil.

The pasta absorbs all the juices in the slow cooker and cooks in the usual way.

19

Chicken and Bean Stew

Non-stick cooking oil spray

900g/2lb skinless chicken breasts

2 x 400g/14oz tinned pinto beans, rinsed & drained

2 x 400g/14oz tinned chopped tomatoes

450g/1lb frozen sweetcorn

350g/12oz salsa, homemade or from a jar

Salt & freshly ground black pepper

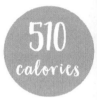

510 calories

- Coat your slow cooker with cooking oil spray. Place the chicken breasts in the slow cooker. Pour the beans over them, then the tomatoes, corn (with juice) and salsa. Season well with salt and pepper.

- Cover and cook on Low for about 7 hours.

- Stir well or use two forks to shred the chicken.

- Serve over cooked brown rice, garnished with fresh parsley, or with tortillas and sour cream.

Black beans or kidney beans also work well with this recipe.

Pulled Cider Chicken

2 eating apples, cored & chopped

1 onion, peeled & finely sliced

1 tsp salt

1 tsp garlic powder

250ml/1 cup cider

900g/2lb skinless chicken breasts or thighs

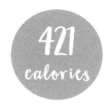
421 calories

- Add the apples and onions to your slow cooker. Season with ½ tsp salt.

- Sprinkle the chicken with the remaining salt and the garlic powder. Add them to the slow cooker, on top of the onion and apples. Pour about ¾ of the cider over the top.

- Cover and cook on High for 4 hours or on Low for 6, until the chicken is very tender.

- Remove the chicken to a chopping board and shred it, using two forks. Return it to the slow cooker, and stir in the rest of the cider.

- Adjust the seasoning or add more cider to taste and serve.

Use dry or sweet cider according to your taste.

Simple Beef Stew

2 tbsp plain flour

½ tsp salt

¼ tsp freshly ground black pepper

675g/1½lb stewing steak, cubed

Non-stick cooking oil spray

1 medium onion, peeled & sliced

1 stalk celery, sliced

450g/1lb tomato passata/sieved tomatoes

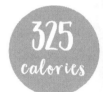

325 calories

- On a plate, mix together the flour, salt and pepper, and lightly coat the steak pieces in the mixture.

- Spray your slow cooker with non-stick oil. Add the onion, floured steak, celery and passata.

- Cover and cook on Low for 8 hours or until the meat is very tender.

- Serve on warmed plates or bowls, garnished with sprigs of freshly picked rosemary. Mop up the juices with some fresh crusty bread.

Stewing steak needs a long, slow cook, so this recipe always works best using the Low heat setting.

Cranberry Brisket

Non-stick cooking oil spray

1.1kg/2½lb boneless beef brisket

Salt & freshly ground black pepper

400g/14oz cranberry sauce

250g/8oz passata/sieved tomatoes

1 onion, peeled & chopped

1 tbsp mustard

349 calories

- Spray the inside of your slow cooker with non-stick oil.

- Rub the brisket all over with plenty of salt and pepper, and place it in the slow cooker.

- In a bowl, mix together the cranberry sauce, passata, onion and mustard. Pour it over the meat.

- Cover and cook on Low for 8-10 hours or until the brisket is very tender.

- Remove the meat from the slow cooker to a serving plate or chopping board. Slice it across the grain.

- With a spoon, skim the fat from cooking juices and discard. To serve, pour the remaining juices over the brisket.

- Optional serving suggestion: Enjoy with boiled new potatoes and steamed greens.

The Cranberry sauce adds sweetness to this lovely beef cut.

Pulled Beef Sandwiches

SERVES 8
SANDWICHES

Non-stick cooking oil spray

1.35kg/3lb boneless brisket or silverside beef

2-3 tbsp chilli seasoning mix

120ml/½ cup barbecue sauce

8 bread rolls, split

8 slices Cheddar cheese

575
calories

- Spray the inside of your slow cooker with non-stick oil.

- Cut the beef in half and place it in the slow cooker. Sprinkle it all over with chilli seasoning. Pour on the barbecue sauce.

- Cover and cook on Low for 8-10 hours, or until the beef is very tender.

- Remove the meat to a chopping board and allow to cool a little. Using two forks, shred the beef. Skim the fat from cooking juices with a spoon, then return the shredded beef to the slow cooker. Cover and leave to warm for another few minutes.

- Split the bread rolls and use a slotted spoon to dollop the meat mixture into each one. Add a slice of cheese to each, close your sandwiches and enjoy with a fresh crispy salad on the side.

This is a delicious (and messy) eating experience the whole family will enjoy.

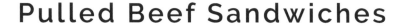

Beef & Mushroom Pasta

Non-stick cooking oil spray

450g/1lb lean stewing steak, cubed

2 carrots, peeled & finely chopped

1 onion, peeled & chopped

2 x 400g/14oz tin cream of mushroom soup

175g/6oz whole wheat pasta

Salt & pepper

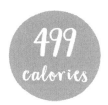

499 calories

- Spray the inside of your slow cooker with non-stick oil. Add in the meat, onions and carrots.

- Combine well and pour the soup over the top.

- Cover and cook on Low for 8 hours, or on High for 4. Stir everything up occasionally.

- About 30 minutes before you wish to serve, stir in the pasta, adding a little water if necessary.

- Adjust the seasoning and serve garnished with parsley and slices of fresh tomato.

If you prefer, cook the pasta separately on the hob, drain and mix into your stew just before you serve.

Beef Fajitas

Non-stick cooking oil spray

450g/1lb salsa

900g/2lbs lean beef, sliced into strips

2 red peppers, deseeded & sliced

1 onion, peeled & finely sliced

2 tbsp fajita seasoning

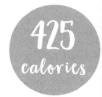

425 calories

- Spray the inside of your slow cooker with non-stick oil. Pour in the salsa, then all the other ingredients. Stir them together to combine well.

- Cover and cook on Low for 7-8 hours, or on High for 3½-4 hours.

- Optional serving suggestion: Serve hot with tortillas or steamed rice, garnished with sour cream.

Add some fresh chillies, lime and avocado when serving for a real Mexican feast.

Easy Chilli Con Carne

1 tbsp olive oil

450g/1lb lean steak mince

400g/14oz tinned chopped tomatoes

225g/8oz passata/sieved

400g/14oz can kidney beans, drained & rinsed

2 tbsp chilli seasoning

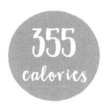

355 calories

- Heat the oil in a pan and brown the mince. Drain it and transfer the meat to your slow cooker.

- Pour in the tomatoes, passata and kidney beans. Sprinkle on the seasoning and stir well to combine.

- Cover and cook on Low for 6 hours.

- Optional serving suggestion: Serve hot over rice, scattered with torn coriander leaves and slivers of fresh chilli.

This recipe also works well with minced turkey.

Beefy Bites

900g/2lb silverside beef, cubed

120ml/½ cup beef stock

1 onion, peeled & finely chopped

2 cloves garlic, crushed

Salt & pepper

60g/2½oz butter

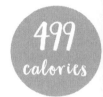

499 calories

- Drop the steak cubes into your slow cooker. Pour the stock over the top. Scatter on the onion and garlic and season well with salt and pepper.

- Dot the butter on top.

- Cover and cook on Low for 7-8 hours or until the meat is very tender.

- Serve warm in bowls, garnished with sprigs of freshly parsley.

- Optional serving suggestion: Crunchy salad and fresh bread on the side.

This simple recipe makes a delicious dinner or a special lunch time snack.

Beef Burritos

Non-stick cooking oil spray

1 onion, peeled & chopped

2 cloves garlic, crushed

900g/2lb boneless silverside, cut in half

1-2 tbsp taco seasoning

1 tbsp balsamic vinegar

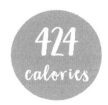

424 calories

- Spray the inside of your slow cooker with non-stick oil.

- Add the onion and garlic to the slow cooker. Rub the two silverside pieces with the taco seasoning and place them on top of the onion. Drizzle the balsamic vinegar over everything.

- Cover and cook on Low for 8 hours. Shred the beef, using two forks.

- Optional serving suggestion: Serve hot with tortillas, and top with slices of avocado and tomato and a light sprinkling of cheese.

Substitute pork shoulder for beef — it's equally delicious.

Beef Ragu

450g/1lb braising steak, cubed

Salt & freshly ground black pepper

10 cloves garlic, peeled & bruised

225g/8oz carrots, chopped

225g/8oz passata/sieved tomatoes

120ml/½ cup red wine

359 calories

- Place the beef in your slow cooker and season well with salt and pepper. Arrange the garlic cloves over the top. Add the carrots.

- In a bowl, whisk together the passata and red wine. Pour the mixture over the meat and vegetables in the slow cooker.

- Cover and cook on Low for 7-8 hours, or on High for 4 hours.

- Stir everything up before serving hot in warmed bowls. Garnish with lots of torn basil and oregano leaves.

- Optional serving suggestion: Serve over whole wheat penne.

To get the best flavour, don't use the cheapest red wine. Use one you would like to drink.

Meatballs

2 x 400g/14oz tinned chopped tomatoes

675g/1½lb beef meatballs

400g/14oz tinned black beans, drained & rinsed

500ml/2 cups beef stock

275g/10oz sweetcorn

Salt & freshly ground black pepper

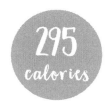

295 calories

- Empty the tomatoes into your slow cooker. Add the meatballs, beans and sweetcorn. Pour the stock in over the top.

- Cover and cook on Low for 6-7 hours or on High for about 3½ hours.

- Optional serving suggestion: Serve hot over rice or pasta, garnished with freshly chopped parsley or oregano.

Make your own meatballs if possible, or use pre-packaged for convenience.

Fruity Pork Chops

SERVES 6

Non-stick cooking oil spray

6 boneless pork loin chops, fat trimmed

Salt and freshly ground black pepper

1 tbsp freshly picked thyme leaves

400g/14oz dried mixed fruits, e.g. prunes and apricots

1 red pepper, de-seeded & sliced

250ml/1 cup barbecue sauce

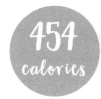

454 calories

- Spray the inside of your slow cooker with non-stick oil. Place the chops in the bottom and season with salt and pepper. Sprinkle them with the thyme. Add the dried fruit and peppers, then pour the barbecue sauce over the top.

- Cover and cook on Low for 4½-5 hours or on High for 2½-3.

- Remove the chops to a serving plate. Skim the fat from sauce and discard. Spoon the sauce over the chops.

- Optional serving suggestion: Serve hot, with new potatoes and crunchy salad. Garnish with fresh sprigs of thyme.

Dried fruit cooks wonderfully in the slow cooker, growing plump and flavoursome!

Glazed Apricot Pork

Non-stick cooking oil spray

250ml/1 cup chicken stock

200g/7oz apricot jam

2 onions, peeled & finely chopped

1 tbsp Dijon mustard

1.1kg/2½lb boneless pork loin

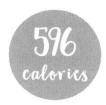

596 calories

- Spray the inside of your slow cooker with non-stick oil.

- In a bowl, mix together the stock, jam, onion, and mustard.

- Place the pork into the slow cooker and pour the stock mix over it.

- Cover and cook on Low for 6 hours, or on High 3-3½ , or until the meat is tender.

- Optional serving suggestion: Serve hot on pre-warmed plates, over rice.

Feel free to substitute other fruit preserves for the apricot.

Pork in Bacon

900g/2lb pork loin, fat trimmed

1 tbsp olive oil

Salt and freshly ground black pepper

1 tbsp fresh oregano, chopped

4 cloves garlic, crushed

1 tbsp brown sugar

6 rashers of back bacon

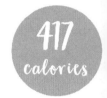
417 calories

- Rub the olive oil over the meat then sprinkle it all over with salt, pepper and oregano. Scatter the garlic and sugar on top of the pork. Drape the bacon rashers over the pork, or wrap them right around if they'll go.

- Place the meat into your slow cooker. Cover and cook on Low for 5 hours.

- Remove the pork and leave to rest for a few minutes. Garnish with sprigs of oregano.

- Optional serving suggestion: Slice and serve with boiled new potatoes and fresh green vegetables.

Thyme instead of oregano also works well with this recipe.

Easy Hawaiian Pork Chops

4 boneless pork chops, fat trimmed

400g/14oz tinned pineapple chunks in juice

1 tbsp brown sugar

½ tsp chilli flakes

1 tbsp soy sauce

Salt and freshly ground black pepper

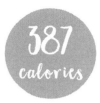

387 calories

- Pour the whole tin of pineapple into your slow cooker. Stir in the sugar, chilli flakes and soy sauce. Place the chops on top and season well with salt and pepper.

- Cover and cook on Low for 6-8 hours or until the meat is tender.

- Optional serving suggestion: Serve hot over rice with a crunchy green salad on the side.

You can also use a fresh pineapple. Juice half of it and add the juice to the slow cooker with the rest cut into chunks.

Pulled Pork

120ml/½ cup beef stock

2 onions, peeled & roughly chopped

900g/2lb boneless pork loin, fat trimmed

Salt and freshly ground black pepper

60ml/¼ cup cider vinegar

1 tsp Worcestershire sauce

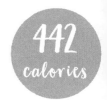

442 calories

- Pour the stock into your slow cooker and stir in the onions.

- Rub the pork evenly with plenty salt and pepper then place it in the slow cooker.

- Cover and cook on Low for 8-9 hours or on High for 4-4½ hours.

- Transfer the pork to a large plate. Remove the onion chunks from the slow cooker with a slotted spoon and add them to the pork. Using two forks, shred the pork.

- In a small bowl, mix together the cider vinegar and Worcestershire sauce. Pour it over the shredded meat and onions. Stir to coat the pork thoroughly.

- Optional serving suggestion: Serve hot in a wrap or baked potato, with crunchy green salad.

Also delicious with beef instead of pork.

Hoisin Pulled Lamb

Non-stick cooking spray

900g/2lb boneless lamb

1 onion, peeled & finely chopped

2 cloves garlic, peeled & crushed

1 tsp of freshly grated ginger

3 tbsp hoisin sauce

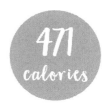

471 calories

- Spray your slow cooker with non-stick oil, then place the lamb inside.

- In a bowl, mix together the onion, garlic, ginger and hoisin sauce. Pour the mixture over the lamb.

- Cover and cook on Low for 8-10 hours or until the lamb is falling-apart tender.

- Remove the lamb to a plate and shred it using 2 forks. Pour the juices over the top, and toss.

- Optional serving suggestion: Serve in wraps or in a fresh, crusty rolls with crunchy salad.

This recipe works well with pork, beef and chicken too.

Italian Roast Pork

Non-stick cooking spray

1 large onion, peeled & roughly chopped

2 tsp Italian salad dressing

900g/2lb boneless rolled pork

1 red pepper, de-seeded and chopped

60ml/¼ cup water

1 courgette, sliced

392 calories

- Spray the inside of your slow cooker with non-stick oil, then add the onions.

- Rub the Italian salad dressing mix evenly over the pork. Place it in the slow cooker with the onion. Add the pepper and water.

- Cover and cook on Low for 8 hours, or on High for 5 hours.

- Add in the courgette, re-cover and cook for another 30 minutes or until the courgette is tender. Remove the meat and the vegetables using a slotted spoon. Skim and discard the fat from the cooking juices and keep warm.

- Slice the meat and serve it with the vegetables on pre-warmed plates. Spoon some cooking liquid over everything to serve.

This is great served with boiled potatoes and fresh basil.

Orange Pork

1 tbsp olive oil

Salt & freshly ground black pepper

900g/2lb shoulder pork

1 tbsp orange marmalade

2 tbsp fresh mint, roughly chopped

1 tbsp fresh parsley, roughly chopped

Zest from ½ lemon, grated

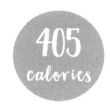

405 calories

- Rub the oil, salt and pepper over the pork. In a small bowl, mix together the marmalade with more black pepper. Spread this over the pork.

- Place the pork in your slow cooker. Cover and cook on Low for 8-9 hours or on High for 4½-5 hours or until the meat is very tender.

- Transfer the pork to a serving plate. Leave it to rest for a few minutes, then shred it, using 2 forks. Spoon a little of the cooking juices over the meat, then sprinkle on the herbs and lemon zest. Mix it all together.

- Optional serving suggestion: Serve with fresh vegetables of your choice.

If you wish to crisp up the crackling on your pork, place it under the grill for a few minutes before you shred it.

Ham and Pineapple

Non-stick cooking spray

900g/2lb boneless ham joint

225g/8oz tinned pineapple chunks, with juice

2 tbsp English mustard

1 tbsp honey

4 cloves garlic, peeled & crushed

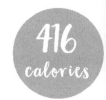

416 calories

- Spray the inside of your slow cooker with non-stick oil.

- Place the ham in the slow cooker.

- In a bowl stir together the pineapple chunks, mustard, honey and garlic. Spread the mixture evenly over the ham.

- Cover and cook on Low for 7-8 hours or until the ham shreds easily.

- Optional serving suggestion: Serve with creamy mashed potato and freshly boiled Chantenay carrots.

Use more or less honey according to your taste.

Ham with Potato and Carrots

450g/1lb boneless ham joint

140g/4½oz whole baby carrots

4 large potatoes, peeled & cubed

500ml/2 cups chicken stock

12 small shallots, peeled

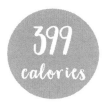

399 calories

- Add the carrots and potatoes into your slow cooker. Place the ham on top of them. Pour the chicken stock over everything.

- Cover and cook on Low for 8 hours.

- Stir in the shallots, re-cover and cook for another 30 minutes or until the shallots are tender.

- Serve hot on pre-warmed plates, garnished with sprigs of fresh parsley or thyme.

Feel free to add in some cabbage or other vegetables, too, but remember it will alter the calorie count!

Herby Lamb with Red Wine

900kg/2lb leg of lamb

Salt & freshly ground black pepper

1 tbsp olive oil

4 large onions, peeled and finely sliced

Small handful of freshly cut thyme sprigs

250ml/1 cup red wine

2 tbsp freshly cut parsley, chopped

520 calories

- Season the lamb well with salt and pepper.

- Spread the olive oil around the inside of your slow cooker. Add the onions and a few sprigs of thyme. Place the lamb on top and pour over the wine.

- Cover and cook on Low for 8-9 hours, or on High for around 4 hours, until the lamb is thoroughly tender.

- Transfer the lamb and onion to a serving plate to rest for a few minutes.

- Mix together the parsley and the leaves of the remaining thyme. Sprinkle them over the lamb.

- Optional serving suggestion: Serve hot on pre-warmed plates, with mint potatoes and fresh spring greens.

Change the herb mixture to suit yourself. For example try with rosemary or sage.

Apricot Lamb Chops

SERVES 4

Non-stick cooking spray

4 medium lamb chops

4 cloves garlic, peeled & crushed

375g/13oz dried apricots, chopped

3 tbsp Dijon mustard

250ml/1 cup red wine

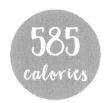

585 calories

- Spray the inside of your slow cooker with non-stick oil.

- Place the lamb chops in the bottom of the slow cooker.

- In a small bowl, stir together the garlic, apricots, and mustard. Spread the mixture all over the chops, then pour the red wine over the top.

- Cover and cook on Low for about 8 hours or on High for 5, until the chops are very tender.

- Garnish with sprigs of rosemary.

- Optional serving suggestion: Serve hot on pre-warmed plates, with creamy mashed potato and leafy green vegetables.

For a stronger mustard flavour, use English mustard instead of Dijon.

Orange and Balsamic Lamb Chops

Non-stick cooking spray

4 medium lamb chops

1 tbsp olive oil, divided

2 tsp grated orange rind

1 tbsp fresh orange juice

3 tbsp balsamic vinegar

Salt and freshly ground black pepper

336 calories

- Spray the inside of your slow cooker with non-stick oil. Place the lamb chops in the slow cooker.

- In a small bowl or jug, mix together the olive oil, orange rind, orange juice and balsamic vinegar. Drizzle the mixture over the top of the chops. Season well with salt and pepper.

- Cover and cook on Low for 7-8 hours or on High for 4, until the lamb is very tender.

- Serve hot on pre-warmed plates with slices of orange.

- Optional serving suggestion: Enjoy with a crispy green salad and fresh bread or boiled new potatoes.

You could use red or white wine vinegar instead of balsamic, but the balsamic imparts a more distinctive and delicious flavour.

Moroccan Lamb Stew

2 tbsp olive oil

4 tbsp Ras El Hanout spice blend

900g/2lb neck of lamb, cubed

2 sweet potatoes, peeled & cubed

1 red pepper, de-seeded & diced

200g/7oz fresh, ripe apricots, stoned & diced

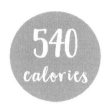

540 calories

- In your slow cooker, combine the oil and Ras El Hanout. Stir in the lamb pieces and coat them thoroughly in the mixture.

- Add in the sweet potatoes, pepper and apricots. Cover and cook on Low for 7-8 hours.

- Serve hot with slices of fresh tomato.

- Optional serving suggestion: Serve over steamed rice.

Use a different cut of lamb if you prefer, but slow cooking works particularly well with cheaper cuts like neck, leaving it tender and flavoursome.

Garlic Roast Lamb

Non-stick cooking spray

500ml/2 cups dry white wine

4 cloves garlic, peeled & crushed

2 tbsp freshly picked parsley, chopped

1½ tsp salt

1.8kg/4lb leg of lamb, on the bone

1 onion, peeled & sliced

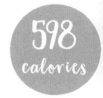

598 calories

- Spray your slow cooker with non-stick oil.

- In a bowl, combine the white wine, garlic, parsley and salt.

- Place the lamb in your slow cooker. Scatter the onion over the lamb and pour the white wine mixture over the top.

- Cover and cook on Low for 8-10 hours, or on High for 5 hours, until the lamb is very tender.

- Transfer to a plate and allow to rest for a few minutes before serving. Carve the lamb and serve garnished with sprigs of fresh mint.

- Optional serving suggestion: Serve with new boiled potatoes and baby carrots.

You'll need a large slow cooker for this recipe, or you could take the meat off the bone prior to cooking.

Easy Lamb Curry

900g/2lb lean boneless lamb, cut into bite-sized cubes

2 tbsp garam masala

675g/1½lb potatoes, peeled and cubed

Salt & freshly ground black pepper

400g/14oz tinned chopped tomatoes with garlic

60ml/¼ cup water

120ml/½ cup natural yogurt

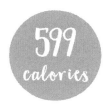

599 calories

- Add the lamb pieces into your slow cooker and sprinkle them with garam masala. Toss to coat the thoroughly in the spice. Season well with salt and pepper. Pour the tomatoes and water over the top.

- Cover and cook on Low for 8-10 hours, or on High for 4-5 hours.

- Just before you serve, stir in the yogurt.

- Optional serving suggestion: Ladle over bowls of rice and top with fresh, shredded coriander leaves.

If you wish, substitute simple curry powder for the garam masala.

Spicy North African Lamb

700g/1lb 9oz lamb, cubed

400g/14oz can chopped tomatoes

2 tsp harissa paste

Salt & freshly ground black pepper

400g/14oz tinned chickpeas, drained & rinsed

2 tbsp fresh coriander, roughly chopped

395 calories

- Add the lamb into your slow cooker along with the tomatoes. Half fill the tomato tin with water and pour it over the top. Add the harissa paste and season well with salt and pepper.

- Cover and cook on Low for 8 hours or on High for 4 or until the lamb is tender.

- Pour in the chickpeas, re-cover and cook for another 30-60 minutes.

- Adjust the seasoning, and then scatter the coriander over the top.

- Serve warm with slices of fresh tomato and a dollop of natural yogurt.

- Optional serving suggestion: add a side serving of couscous.

Feel free to use the cheapest cuts of lamb since slow cooking it makes it beautifully tender.

Mint-Glazed Lamb

SERVES 6

Non-stick cooking spray

1 onion, finely sliced

900g/2lb boneless leg of lamb

3 tbsp mint jelly

10 freshly picked mint leaves, roughly chopped

4 cloves garlic, peeled & finely chopped

Salt & freshly ground black pepper

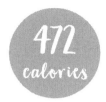

472 calories

- Spray the inside of your slow cooker with non-stick oil.

- Add the onions into your slow cooker, and place the lamb on top.

- In a small bowl, mix together the mint jelly, fresh mint and garlic. Season well with salt, and pepper. Spread the mixture all over the lamb.

- Cover and cook on Low for 7-8 hours or until the lamb is tender.

- Serve hot on pre-warmed plates and spoon some of the cooking juices over the top. Garnish with sprigs of fresh rosemary.

- Optional serving suggestion: Enjoy with mashed potatoes and spring greens.

The mint glaze is perfect for lamb but also works well with beef and game meats.

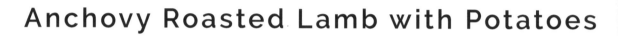

Anchovy Roasted Lamb with Potatoes

581 calories

Non-stick cooking spray

100g/3½oz jar anchovies in olive oil

4 cloves garlic, peeled

1 tbsp mint sauce

900g/2lb boneless leg of lamb

4 medium potatoes, unpeeled & cut into wedges

Salt & freshly ground black pepper

- Spray the inside of your slow cooker with non-stick oil.

- Empty the jar of anchovies into a food processor. Add the garlic and the mint sauce and blend to a smooth paste. Spread the paste all over the lamb.

- Arrange the potato slices on the bottom of the slow cooker, and place the lamb on top.

- Cover and cook on Low for 8 hours, or on High for 4 or 5 or until the lamb is tender all the way through.

- Serve with sprigs of fresh mint.

- Optional serving suggestion: Add a side serving of baby carrots.

Anchovies add depth of flavour to this tasty meal!

Skinny
SLOW COOKER
fish dishes

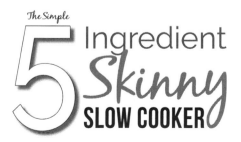

The Simple
5 Ingredient Skinny
SLOW COOKER

Salmon & Rice

1 tbsp butter

1 onion, peeled & chopped

1 red pepper, de-seeded & chopped

500ml/2 cups vegetable stock

150g/5oz rice

4 fresh salmon fillets each weighing 150g/5oz

Salt & freshly ground black pepper

525 calories

- Turn your slow cooker on to High and drop in the butter. When it begins to melt, stir in the onion and pepper, then pour in the stock.

- Cover and cook on High for 30 minutes.

- Stir in the rice, cover and cook for a further 15 minutes.

- Season the salmon with salt and pepper and lay the fillets on top of the rice.

- Cover once more and cook for another hour.

- Serve on warmed plates, garnished with freshly cut sprigs of parsley and a few drops of fresh lime juice. Enjoy with a crisp green salad on the side.

This simple recipe is also delicious with other varieties of fish.

Coley Chowder

1 tbsp olive oil

1 onion, peeled & chopped

4 medium potatoes, peeled & cubed

120ml/½ cup dry white wine

400g/14oz tinned chopped tomatoes with garlic

2 smoked coley fillets each weighing 150g/5oz

358 calories

- Pour the olive oil into your slow cooker and spread it around. Stir in the onions, then pour in the wine and the tomatoes with their juice.

- Cover and cook on High for an hour.

- Lay the coley fillets on top of the vegetables. Re-cover and cook on High for another 1½-2 hours or until the potatoes are soft and the fish breaks easily against a fork.

- Stir everything together and serve garnished with sprigs of freshly cut parsley.

- Optional serving suggestion: Enjoy on its own or with warm crusty bread or pasta.

For a non-alcoholic version, use chicken stock or water instead of wine.

Garlic Salmon with Dill

490
calories

2 tbsp olive oil

4 onions, peeled & chopped

450g/1lb baby carrots, whole

4 cloves garlic, peeled & crushed

675g/1½lb salmon fillet

Salt & freshly ground black pepper

7g/¼oz freshly picked dill, chopped

- Pour the olive oil into hour slow cooker. Add the onions, garlic & carrots and combine well.

- Cover and cook on Low for 3-4 hours, stirring once if you can during cooking.

- Place the salmon fillet on top of the vegetables. Season with salt and pepper, and scatter the dill over the top.

- Cover and cook on Low for another hour or 2; until the salmon flakes against a fork.

- To serve, place the salmon on a platter and pour the onion mixture over the top.

- Enjoy with sweet cherry tomatoes and a crunchy salad.

You could use four small salmon fillets instead of the larger piece, but don't cook for longer than an hour.

Tilapia with Garlic Butter

1 tbsp butter
2 cloves garlic, peeled & crushed
1 tbsp fresh parsley, chopped
4 tilapia fillets each weighing 150g/5oz
Salt & freshly ground black pepper
Juice of ½ fresh lemon

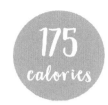

175 calories

- In a bowl, mash together the butter, garlic and parsley.

- Place a sheet of aluminium foil in your slow cooker. Place the tilapia fillets onto it. Season the fish well with salt and pepper. Divide the garlic butter evenly between the fillets. Drizzle lemon juice over the top, and wrap the foil around the fish.

- Cover and cook on High for 2 hours.

- Unwrap the foil with care, and serve the fish with the juices poured over the top. Garnish with a slice of lemon and a fresh sprig of parsley.

- Optional serving suggestion: Enjoy with green vegetables and herby new potatoes.

This is a great recipe for when you're not out of the kitchen for too long — don't cook it for longer than 2 hours.

Thai Shrimp Curry

750ml/3 cups light coconut milk

120ml/½ cup Thai red curry paste

2½ tsp lemon pepper seasoning

1 tbsp fresh coriander, chopped

600g/1lb 5oz king prawns, with shells

386 calories

- Pour the coconut milk into your slow cooker. Stir in the red curry paste, lemon pepper and half the coriander.

- Cover and cook on High for 2 hours.

- Add the shrimp and the rest of the coriander, re-cover and cook for a further 20-30 minutes or until the shrimp are cooked.

- Serve hot over brown rice or couscous, garnished with fresh coriander leaves, desiccated coconut and a spoonful of natural yogurt.

Test the shrimp frequently after 10 minutes cooking — you may find they cook faster than expected.

Tarragon Salmon

900g/2lb salmon fillets
Salt & freshly ground black pepper
2 cloves garlic, crushed
1 tbsp fresh tarragon, chopped
1 fresh lemon, sliced
1 tbsp olive oil

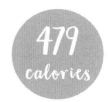

479 calories

- Line your slow cooker with parchment. Lay the salmon on top, and season well with salt, pepper, garlic and tarragon. Arrange the lemon slices on the fish and drizzle the oil over the top.

- Cover and cook on High for 1-2 hours or until the salmon flakes against a fork.

- Lift out the parchment and serve the salmon.

- Optional serving suggestion: Serve on a bed of rice and courgettes.

Chopped dill also works well with this recipe in place of tarragon.

Pesto Sole

900g/2lb fresh Dover sole fillets

2 tbsp pesto

2 tsp Parmesan cheese, grated

2 courgettes, sliced

4 spears fresh asparagus

198 calories

- Spread out a small sheet of foil. Place a piece of fish on it. Spread on a teaspoon of pesto. Add a couple of slices of courgette and an asparagus spear then sprinkle a little Parmesan over the top.

- Fold over the foil to make a parcel and put it in your slow cooker. Repeat with each fillet

- Cover and cook on Low for 2-3 hours until the fish flakes against a fork.

- Unwrap the parcels carefully and serve immediately with crusty bread to mop up the juices.

Lemon sole will work too if you can't get Dover sole.

Trout in White Wine

Non-stick cooking spray

4 fresh medium whole trout, gutted & headed

125g/4oz mushrooms, sliced

180ml/¾ cup white wine

Juice & grated rind of 1 lemon

Salt & freshly ground black pepper

120ml/½ cup creme fraiche

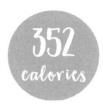

352 calories

- Spray the inside of your slow cooker with non-stick oil.

- Arrange the trout in the slow cooker. Add the mushrooms, wine, and the lemon rind and juice. Season with salt and pepper.

- Cover and cook on Low for 3 to 4 hours.

- Stir in the creme fraiche and heat a further 15 minutes or so.

- Optional serving suggestion: Serve warm with new potatoes, and steamed fresh green vegetables.

It's easy to overcook fish, so to be safe, check it after 2 hours. Slow cookers may vary!

Cod in Tomato Sauce

168 calories

SERVES 4

400g/14oz tinned chopped tomatoes with garlic

1 tbsp tomato puree

Salt & freshly ground black pepper

1 green pepper, de-seeded & diced

1 onion, peeled & finely chopped

4 cod steaks (each weighing 150g/5oz each)

- In a bowl, stir together the chopped tomatoes and tomato puree. Season with salt and pepper. Stir in the green pepper and onion.

- Place the fish steaks in your slow cooker and pour the tomato sauce over the top.

- Cover and cook on Low for 2 to 3 hours, or on High for around 1-2.

- Serve with slices of fresh tomato and cucumber. Garnish with torn fresh basil leaves.

For this recipe, you can substitute any firm white fish for the cod.

Skinny
SLOW COOKER
vegetable &
vegetarian dishes

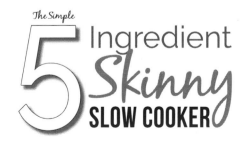

The Simple
5 Ingredient
Skinny
SLOW COOKER

Stuffed Peppers

4 fresh peppers, any colour will do

400g/14oz tinned baked beans with chilli

250g/8oz cooked rice

225g/4oz Cheddar cheese, grated

Salt & freshly ground black pepper

400g/14oz passata/sieved tomatoes

379 calories

- Cut the tops off the peppers and de-seed them. Reserve the tops.

- In a bowl, stir together the chilli beans, rice, and half of the cheese. Season with salt and pepper. Spoon the mixture into the peppers and replace the tops.

- Pour the passata into your slow cooker. Place the filled peppers in the sauce.

- Cover and cook on Low for 6-6½ hours or on High for 3-3½.

- Transfer the peppers to a serving plate. Spoon the tomato sauce over the peppers and scatter the remaining cheese on top.

Instead of chilli beans, try with chickpeas and a couple of cloves of crushed garlic.

Linguine with Artichoke

Non-stick cooking spray

2 x 400g/14oz tinned chopped tomatoes with garlic

2 x 400g/14oz cans artichoke hearts, drained & quartered

6 cloves garlic, peeled & crushed

120ml/½ cup double cream

350g/12oz dried linguine

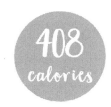

- Spray the inside of your slow cooker with non-stick oil.

- Pour the chopped tomatoes into the slow cooker. Add the artichoke hearts and the garlic.

- Cover and cook on Low for 6-8 hours or on High for 3-4 hours.

- Stir in the cream and leave to heat through for about 5 minutes.

- Cook the pasta separately, according to the packet instructions, and drain.

- Serve the sauce over the pasta in pre-warmed bowls. Garnish with olives and Parmesan cheese.

To lower the calorie count a little more, use crème fraiche or low fat natural yogurt instead of double cream.

Cajun Vegetable Casserole

2 x 400g/14oz tinned black beans, rinsed & drained

2 x 400g/14oz tinned tomatoes

2 onions, peeled & chopped

1 tbsp Cajun seasoning

151 calories

- In your slow cooker stir together the beans, tomatoes, onions and Cajun seasoning.

- Cover and cook on Low for 6-8 hours or on High for 3-4 hours.

- Optional serving suggestion: Serve hot over cooked brown rice and scatter with torn basil leaves.

Feel free to vary the vegetables you use according to what you have in your kitchen.

Sweetcorn Chowder

3 medium potatoes, peeled & cubed

2 x 400g/14oz tinned creamed sweetcorn

200g/7oz tinned sweetcorn

Salt and freshly ground black pepper

500g/2 cups vegetable stock

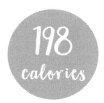

198 calories

- In your slow cooker, stir together the potatoes, cream-style corn and sweetcorn. Season well with salt and a lot of black pepper. Pour in the stock.

- Cover and cook on Low for 6-8 hours or on High for 3-4 hours.

- Ladle into bowls sand scatter with torn coriander leaves and freshly ground black pepper.

- Optional serving suggestion: Enjoy with warm, crusty bread

This is great with a little green chilli added to the slow cooker too.

Vegetable Roast

2 tbsp olive oil

2 peppers, any colours, de-seeded & roughly chopped

1 large sweet potato, peeled & cubed

3 small courgettes, roughly chopped

4 whole fresh garlic cloves, peeled

Salt & freshly ground black pepper

Handful of fresh basil leaves, torn

144 calories

- Pour the olive oil into your slow cooker and spread it around. Tip in all the vegetables and stir everything up to coat in the oil. Season with the salt and pepper and sprinkle in the basil.

- Cook on Low for about 6 hours or on High for 3 hours. If you're around, give the vegetables an occasional stir.

- Strain the vegetables into a serving bowl, and serve garnished with fresh herbs. Enjoy as a meal on its own or as accompaniment to another dish.

When you strain the vegetables, save the liquid for stock or just for a delicious veggie drink!

Lentil Curry

1 tsp coconut oil

1 onion, finely chopped

6 cloves garlic, peeled & crushed

1 tbsp curry powder

Salt & freshly ground black pepper

400g/14oz light coconut milk

400g/14oz green lentils, uncooked, well-rinsed

750ml/3 cups boiling water

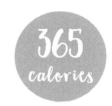

365 calories

- Heat the coconut oil in a small pan. Add the onion and garlic and cook gently for about 5 minutes, stirring occasionally. Add the curry powder, salt and pepper and stir for another half minute or so.

- Scrape the mixture into your slow cooker. Stir in the coconut milk, lentils and water.

- Cover and cook on Low for 7-8 hours or on High for about 4.

- Garnish with chopped fresh coriander leaves and spring onions.

- Optional serving suggestion: Serve over brown rice or couscous.

You can store leftovers in the fridge for up to 3 days, or in the freezer for up to 3 months in an airtight container.

Macaroni Cheese

1 tbsp butter, diced

300g/11oz dried macaroni

225g/8oz mature Cheddar cheese, grated

125g/4oz Gruyere cheese, grated

500ml/2 cups semi-skimmed milk

Salt & freshly ground black pepper

538 calories

- Drop the butter into your slow cooker. Tip in the macaroni and stir to coat the pasta. Stir in both varieties of cheese and pour in the milk. Season well, then stir everything up.

- Cover and cook on Low for about 5 hours, stirring occasionally until the pasta is tender.

- Serve hot in pre-warmed pasta bowls, garnished with fresh basil and parsley, and sprinkled with Parmesan and more black pepper. Enjoy with a crunchy salad on the side, or as an accompaniment to another dish.

Vary your cheeses to find the combination you like best.

Broccoli with Tortellini Marinara

750g/1lb 11oz jar marinara pasta sauce

60ml/¼ cup water

1 tbsp fresh basil leaves, torn

1 tbsp fresh oregano, chopped

Salt and freshly ground black pepper

250g/9oz pre-packed spinach and cheese tortellini

450g/1lb fresh broccoli, broken into florets

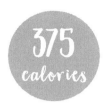

375 calories

- In a bowl, combine the marinara sauce, water basil and oregano. Season well with salt and pepper.

- Pour about a third of the sauce into your slow cooker, then tip in the tortellini. Pour half the remaining sauce over the tortellini. Distribute the broccoli over the top and pour on the remaining sauce.

- Cover and cook on High for 2-2½ hours, until the broccoli and pasta are tender but not mushy.

- Serve hot in pasta bowls, with slices of ripe tomato and freshly picked parsley and basil to garnish.

Use a different pasta sauce if you prefer. For best results make your own, but for ease, there are several varieties easily available in supermarkets.

Aubergine Ragu

226 calories

2 tbsp olive oil

1 large onion, peeled & chopped

1 large aubergine, peeled, cut into 1-inch pieces

Salt and freshly ground black pepper

5 cloves garlic, peeled & crushed

2 x 400g/14oz tinned tomatoes

7g/¼oz fresh basil leaves, torn

- Pour the oil into your slow cooker. Tip in the onion and aubergine and season with salt and pepper. Stir everything up to coat the vegetables.

- Stir in the garlic, tomatoes and basil.

- Cover and cook on Low for 4-5 hours or on High for 3, until the aubergine is tender.

- Garnish with fresh basil leaves and grated Parmesan.

- Optional serving suggestion: Serve over brown rice , pasta or polenta.

Use this basic recipe with any vegetables you like, for example carrots and courgettes.

Sugar-Glazed Carrots

Non-stick cooking spray

1 onion, peeled & finely chopped

900g/2lb fresh whole baby carrots

Salt & freshly ground black pepper

1 tbsp brown sugar

1 tbsp butter

1 tbsp chopped fresh parsley

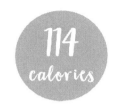

114 calories

- Spray the inside of your slow cooker with non-stick oil.

- Tip in the onion and carrots. Sprinkle them with salt, brown sugar and butter.

- Cover and cook on High for about 4 hours, stirring once if you can, until the carrots are as tender as you like them.

- Transfer the carrot and onion with their juices into a serving bowl. Season with additional salt and pepper and sprinkle with the parsley.

- Serve warm as an accompaniment to a main dish, or cold as a salad.

The sugar gives the carrots an attractive glaze, but feel free to omit the sugar if you find the carrot and onion combination sweet enough without.

Skinny
SLOW COOKER
soups

The Simple
5 Ingredient
Skinny
SLOW COOKER

Pea and Ham Soup

1.25lt/5 cups chicken stock

1 ham hock (weighing approx. 1.3kg/3lb)

550g/1¼lb split peas, dried

1 onion, peeled & chopped

3 carrots, peeled & chopped

Salt & freshly ground black pepper

361 calories

- Trim the hock and place the ham in your slow cooker along with the vegetables. Season with salt and pepper. Pour in the stock and stir everything together.

- Cover and cook on Low for 8 hours, or in High for 4, until the vegetables are tender.

- Remove the ham hock from the slow cooker and slice up the meat. Return the chunks to the soup and leave to warm again for a few minutes.

- Serve hot in bowls, garnished with sprigs of freshly cut parsley and a swirl of yogurt. Enjoy with warm, crusty bread.

Instead of a whole ham hock, which gives the fullest flavour, you can use pieces of ham.

Cream of Asparagus Soup

900g/2lbs fresh asparagus, trimmed
1 onion, peeled & chopped
1 clove garlic, peeled & crushed
1.25lt/5 cups vegetable stock
Salt and freshly ground black pepper
120ml/½ cup double cream

121 calories

- Tip the asparagus, onion and garlic into your slow cooker. Season with salt and pepper and pour in the stock.

- Cover and cook on Low for 6-8 hours, or on High for 3-4.

- Blend the soup until smooth. Stir in the cream and serve hot with sprigs of fresh mint or parsley. Swirl in a little extra cream if you wish.

This is still delicious simply using water instead of stock.

Easy Burger Soup

326 calories

2 x 1lt cartons vegetable juice, e.g. V8

1 onion, peeled & chopped

450g/1lb frozen mixed vegetables

225g/8oz lean steak mince, cooked & drained

300g/11oz tin condensed cream of mushroom soup

Salt and freshly ground black pepper

- Pour the vegetable juice into your slow cooker. Stir in the onion, mixed vegetables, mince and mushroom soup.

- Cover and cook on Low for 7-8 hours, or on High for around 4.

- Season with salt and pepper to taste, and serve hot in pre-warmed bowls. Garnish with finely chopped spring onions.

This is a great way to use up left over mince. Or plan ahead when you have a mince recipe for dinner, and cook half a pound extra for making soup the next day.

Butternut Squash Soup

1 onion, peeled & chopped

3 carrots, peeled & chopped

1 butternut squash, peeled, de-seeded & cubed

1 apple, peeled, cored & chopped

1lt/4 cups vegetable stock

Salt & freshly ground black pepper, to taste

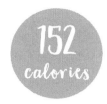

152 calories

- Tip the onion, carrots, squash and apple into your slow cooker. Pour in the stock and stir.

- Cook on Low for 6 hours, or on High for about 3½, until the vegetables are tender.

- Blend the soup until smooth. Season well with salt and pepper to taste.

- Ladle into pre-warmed bowls and serve sprinkled with ground nutmeg and cinnamon. Swirl in a little cream for added decadence!

A delicious autumn and winter soup. Try also with pumpkin instead of squash.

Easy Pasta Soup

450g/1lb tomato pasta sauce

1lt/4 cups of chicken stock

400g/14oz tinned cannellini beans, drained & rinsed

60g/2½oz fresh baby spinach

75g/3oz dried pasta

Salt & freshly ground black pepper

152 calories

- Pour the pasta sauce and chicken stock into your slow cooker. Stir in the beans and the spinach.

- Cover and cook on Low for about 7 hours, or on High for 3-4.

- Stir in the pasta, re-cover and cook for another 30 minutes or until the pasta is tender. Adjust the seasoning.

- Serve hot, garnished with torn basil leaves, and enjoy with warm, crusty bread.

A great, tasty soup to throw together when you're short on time. Use your favourite jar/tub of pasta sauce, or preferably your own home-made tomato sauce.

Chorizo Soup

1lt/4 cups vegetable stock
400g/14oz tinned chopped tomatoes
450g/1lb uncooked chorizo sausage
450g/1lb kale, stems cut off & roughly chopped
4 cloves garlic, peeled & crushed

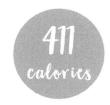

411 calories

- Pour the vegetable stock into your slow cooker. Stir in the tomatoes, chorizo, kale and garlic.

- Cover and cook on Low for 6-8 hours, or on High for 3-4.

- Serve hot in pre-warmed bowls, sprinkled with grated parmesan and a few torn coriander leaves.

Try also with other green veg instead of kale, e.g. spinach, broccoli or cabbage.

Ham and Bean Soup

1lt/4 cups vegetable stock
1 ham hock (weighing approx. 1.3kg/3lb)
450g/1lb tinned pinto beans, drained & rinsed
1 onion, peeled & chopped
175ml/6floz passata/sieved tomatoes
Salt and freshly ground black pepper

392 calories

- Pour the stock into your slow cooker. Add the ham, beans and onions. If necessary pour in some more boiling water to cover the ham.

- Cover and cook on Low for 8 hours, or on High for 5.

- Take the ham out of the slow cooker and shred the meat off the bone. Tip the shredded meat back into the soup.

- Stir in the passata and season to taste.

- Serve hot, garnished with sprigs of fresh parsley. Enjoy with a crisp green salad.

Be sure to taste the soup before you season. With ham, you may find it's salty enough.

Mexican Chicken Soup

Cooking spray

4 fresh chicken breasts (each weighing 150g/5oz)

1 tbsp taco seasoning

225g/8oz salsa

2lt/4 cups chicken stock

400g/14oz tinned black beans, drained & rinsed

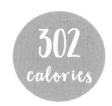

302 calories

- Spray the inside of your slow cooker with non-stick oil.

- Place the chicken in the bottom of the slow cooker. Sprinkle the taco seasoning over the top. Pour on the salsa and the chicken stock, then stir in the beans.

- Cover and cook on Low for 8-10 hours, or on High for 5-6, until the chicken is very tender.

- Using a slotted spoon, take out the chicken breasts and shred them with 2 forks. Return the shredded chicken to the soup and stir.

- Re-cover and cook for another 30 minutes before serving.

Serve hot, garnished with torn coriander leaves, finely chopped garlic, a sprinkling of cheese and a slice of lime.

Fresh Tomato Soup

131 calories

1 tbsp olive oil
1 large carrot, peeled & chopped
1 stalk celery
1 onion, peeled & chopped
Salt & freshly ground black pepper
900g/2lbs ripe tomatoes, chopped
250ml/1 cup vegetable stock

- Heat the olive oil in a pan and sauté the carrots, celery and onion with some salt and pepper.

- Tip them into your slow cooker. Add the tomatoes and pour in the stock.

- Cover and cook on Low for 5-7 hours, or on High for about 3½.

- Blend the soup until smooth.

- Adjust the seasoning and serve hot sprinkled with chopped fresh basil and oregano and a twist or two of freshly ground black pepper.

If you prefer your soup chunky, blend only half of it.

Simple Lentil Soup

2 tbsp olive oil

1 onion, peeled & finely chopped

400g/14oz tinned chopped tomatoes

225g/8oz red lentils, rinsed

1lt/4 cups vegetable stock

Salt & freshly ground black pepper

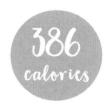
386 calories

- Turn your slow cooker on to High. Pour in the olive oil and spread it around. Stir in the onion for a few minutes, then add the tomatoes, lentils and stock.

- Cover and cook on High for 2 hours. Reduce to Low and cook for a further 7 hours.

- Adjust the seasoning and ladle into bowls. Garnish with sprigs of fresh parsley, and enjoy with warm, crusty bread.

Feel free to add any vegetables or herbs you like to this basic recipe.

Skinny
SLOW COOKER
treats & puddings

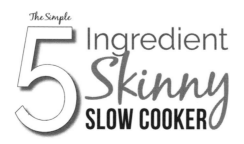

Chocolate Fudge

350g/12oz milk chocolate chips
60ml/¼ cup double cream
125g/4oz honey
60g/2½oz white chocolate chips
1 tsp vanilla extract

SERVES 6

386 calories

- Tip the milk chocolate chips into your slow cooker. Pour in the cream and honey.

- Cover and cook on High for an hour.

- Stir in the white chocolate chips until they melt. Then stir in the vanilla.

- Pour the mixture into a lined baking dish. Leave to cool completely for 2-3 hours, then cut into squares.

- Serve as a snack in small bowls sprinkled with icing sugar and sprigs of fresh mint.

You're unlikely to have any of these left over, but if you do, don't store them in the fridge but at room temperature in an airtight container.

Cherry Pudding

Non-stick cooking spray

1 packet vanilla cake mix

2 x 400g/14oz tins black cherry fruit filling

125g/4oz butter

A few fresh cherries to serve

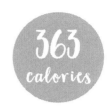

363 calories

- Spray the inside of your slow cooker with non-stick oil.

- Empty the fruit filling into the bottom of your slow cooker, and spread it out evenly.

- In a bowl, stir together the vanilla cake mix and the melted butter. When it's crumbly, pour it over the fruit in the slow cooker. Spread it out evenly.

- Cover and cook on Low for 4 hours, or on High for 2.

- Serve in dessert bowls with a few fresh cherries on top.

- Optional serving suggestion: Add a scoopful of whipped cream or ice cream.

Any fruity pie-filling, including lemon or lime meringue pie filling, will work with this simple recipe.

Peach Cobbler

288
calories

Non-stick cooking spray

900g/1lb fresh or frozen ripe peaches, peeled & sliced

50g/2oz light brown sugar, plus 100g/3½oz

½ tsp ground cinnamon, plus ½ tsp

1 packet vanilla cake mix

60ml/¼ cup milk

- Spray your slow cooker with non-stick oil.

- In a bowl, mix together 50g/2oz sugar and ½ tsp cinnamon. Stir in the peaches to coat thoroughly, then arrange them on the bottom of the slow cooker.

- In another bowl, stir together the cake mix, the rest of the sugar and cinnamon, and the milk. Make sure there are no lumps, then spread the mixture over the peaches in the slow cooker.

- Cover, with a tea towel trapped under the lid to catch condensation drips, and cook on Low for about 4 hours, or until the centre of the dessert is set.

- Serve hot or cold with a sprig of fresh mint. Sprinkle a little fresh ground nutmeg over the top.

You can use a little more or less cinnamon in this recipe, according to your taste.

Cranberry Scones

225g/8oz self-raising flour

Pinch salt

25g/1oz caster sugar

50g/2oz butter cubed

120ml/½ cup semi-skimmed milk

100g/3½oz dried cranberries

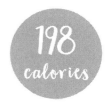

198 calories

- In a bowl, combine the flour, salt and sugar. Rub in the butter, then stir in the milk to make a soft dough. Stir in the dried cranberries. Gently form the dough into a round shape.

- Line your slow cooker, and carefully place the round inside.

- Cover, with a tea towel trapped under the lid to catch drips of condensation, and cook on High for about 1½-2 hours, until a skewer comes out of the cake clean.

- Take the cake out of the slow cooker and leave to cool. Slice it into 8 scones and serve.

- Optional serving suggestion: Enjoy with butter, sugar, jam or cream.

Use dried cherries, blueberries, chocolate chips or any other filling you like instead of the dried cranberries.

Creamy Fudge

Non-stick cooking spray

275g/10oz caster sugar

100g/3½oz golden syrup

225g/8oz clotted cream

½ tsp vanilla extract

436 calories

- Spray your slow cooker with non-stick oil.

- Pour the sugar, syrup, cream and vanilla into the slow cooker and stir everything together.

- Cover and cook on Low for 4 hours.

- Stir it every 10 minutes or so. Once cooked, the fudge will look thin and shiny. Whisk it until it thickens.

- Pour the fudge into a baking tin to cool and set. Then cut into squares, ready to eat.

If you can, substitute a natural sweetener like Sukrin Gold for the brown sugar. It will bring the calorie count down below 300.

Stuffed Apples

4 sweet & crispy apples, e.g. gala

250g/9oz granola

2 tbsp melted butter

4 tsp maple syrup

½ tsp ground cinnamon

353 calories

- Slice a "lid" off the top of the apples. Using a spoon or a corer, scrape out the core and seeds from each.

- Fill each apple with granola and place it in the slow cooker.

- Drizzle the melted butter and maple syrup over the apples.

- Cover, and cook on High for 2-2½ hours until the apples are tender, but not soft enough to fall apart.

- Serve sprinkled with cinnamon and cloves.

Make this as dessert with a main meal, or as a special breakfast.

Triple Chocolate Pudding

SERVES 8

1 packet chocolate cake mix

1 packet chocolate pudding mix

300g/11oz Nutella

360ml/12½floz semi-skimmed milk

225g/4oz butter, melted

525 calories

- Line your slow cooker with parchment.

- Spread the dry cake mix evenly on the bottom, then spread the pudding mix on top. Drizzle the melted butter and the milk evenly over everything. Spread the Nutella over the top.

- Cover and cook on Low for 3-4 hours, until the centre is still a little gooey but the sides of the cake are firm.

- Remove the cake from the slow cooker, slice and enjoy hot or cold, with cream or ice cream and fresh cherries.

Try also with different chocolate spreads or sauces instead of Nutella.

Glazed Pecans

SERVES 12

Non-stick cooking spray

400g/14oz pecan nuts

1 medium egg white

2 tsp vanilla extract

200g/7oz brown sugar

1½ tbsp ground cinnamon

60ml/¼ cup water

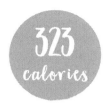

323 calories

- Spray the inside of your slow cooker with non-stick oil.

- Tip the pecans inside.

- In a small bowl, whisk together the egg white and vanilla extract until it foams. Pour the mixture over the nuts and stir to coat them evenly.

- In another bowl, mix the sugar with the cinnamon. Sprinkle it over the pecans and stir to coat all the nuts.

- Cover and cook on Low for 3 hours, stirring every 20 minutes or so. In the last 20 minutes, stir in the water.

- At the end of cooking, empty the nuts in a single layer onto parchment to cool.

- Serve in bowls with a few shakes of salt.

Use this recipe also with peanuts, almonds or cashew nuts.

Caramel Apple Dip with Shortbread

SERVES 6

Non-stick cooking spray

3 eating apples, peeled, cored & chopped

250g/8oz caramel sauce

½ tsp ground cinnamon

Pinch nutmeg

12 shortbread biscuits

281 calories

- Spray your slow cooker with non-stick oil.

- In the slow cooker, stir together the apples, caramel sauce, cinnamon and nutmeg, until the apples are thoroughly coated.

- Cover and cook on High for about 2 hours.

- Pour the mixture out into a bowl and serve

- Optional serving suggestion: Serve with a plate of shortbread for dipping in the apples.

Try this sauce with other butter biscuits, puff pastry or popcorn.

Easy Chocolate Brownies

Non-stick cooking spray

1 packet chocolate brownie cake mix

125g/4oz butter, melted

60ml/¼ cup water, plus 175ml/6floz

2 eggs

350g/12oz fudge sauce

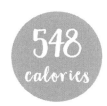

548 calories

- Spray your slow cooker with non-stick oil.

- In a bowl, whisk together the brownie mix, butter, 60ml/¼ cup water, and the eggs. Pour the mixture into the slow cooker.

- In another bowl whisk the fudge sauce into 175ml/6floz hot water. Pour it over the brownie mix in the slow cooker.

- Cover and cook on High for about 3 hours, or until the edges are firm and the centre slightly gooey.

- Slice into large squares.

Make your own fudge sauce for this recipe, or simply use a store-bought one for ease.

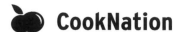 **CookNation**

Other CookNation titles

If you enjoyed 'The Simple 5 Ingredient *Skinny* Slow Cooker Recipe Book' you may also enjoy other books from CookNation including:

'The *Skinny* Slow Cooker Recipe Book'

'The *Skinny* 5:2 Recipe Book'

'The *Skinny* 30 Minute Meals'

To browse the extensive calorie counted '*Skinny*' range and other food & drink books books visit **www.bellmackenzie.com**

Printed in Great Britain
by Amazon